Table Of Contents

I0792257

Chapter 1: Introduction to Moringa

The Origins of Moringa

The origins of moringa, often referred to as the "miracle tree," can be traced back to the Himalayan region of India, where it has been cultivated for thousands of years. Moringa oleifera, the most well-known species, is revered for its remarkable nutritional profile and medicinal properties. This tree thrives in various climates, particularly in tropical and subtropical regions, which has facilitated its spread across Africa, Asia, and Latin America. Its adaptability to diverse environmental conditions has made it a valuable resource for communities seeking sustainable food and health solutions.

As a vital component of traditional medicine, moringa has been utilized for centuries by various cultures for its health benefits. In India, Ayurvedic practitioners have long recognized moringa's therapeutic properties, employing its leaves, pods, and seeds to treat ailments ranging from inflammation to digestive issues. The leaves are particularly noted for their high concentrations of vitamins, minerals, and antioxidants, making them an essential part of many traditional diets. Similarly, African cultures have harnessed the tree's potential to combat malnutrition and support overall health, incorporating moringa into local culinary practices and remedies.

Moringa's importance extends beyond its nutritional and medicinal uses; it also plays a significant role in environmental sustainability. The tree's fast growth rate and ability to thrive in poor soil conditions make it an ideal candidate for agroforestry systems. Moringa not only provides food and medicinal benefits but also helps improve soil quality and combat desertification. Its deep root system aids in water retention, which is crucial in arid regions. As communities increasingly recognize the need for sustainable agricultural practices, moringa is becoming a focal point in efforts to enhance food security and promote ecological balance.

In addition to its health and environmental benefits, moringa oil has gained attention for its applications in beauty and skincare. Extracted from the seeds of the moringa tree, this oil is rich in oleic acid and antioxidants, making it a popular choice for natural beauty products. It is known for its moisturizing properties and ability to nourish the skin, promoting a healthy complexion. With the growing demand for natural and organic beauty solutions, moringa oil has found its place in various formulations, appealing to health enthusiasts and those seeking cruelty-free alternatives.

The comprehensive benefits of moringa underscore its significance in contemporary health and wellness discussions. As research continues to unveil the myriad advantages of this remarkable tree, its applications in herbal remedies and natural healing are becoming increasingly relevant. For parents and caregivers, moringa presents a valuable option for enhancing nutrition and supporting the well-being of children. The tree's rich array of nutrients and health benefits makes it an ideal addition to the diets of vegans and vegetarians, further solidifying moringa's place as a cornerstone in the pursuit of sustainable wellness.

Nutritional Profile of Moringa

Moringa, often referred to as the "Miracle Tree," boasts an impressive nutritional profile that appeals to health enthusiasts and wellness seekers alike. This plant is a powerhouse of essential nutrients, including vitamins, minerals, and amino acids. Moringa leaves are particularly rich in vitamins A, C, and E, which play a crucial role in promoting healthy skin, boosting the immune system, and combating oxidative stress. The high concentration of these vitamins makes moringa an invaluable addition to a balanced diet, especially for those pursuing plant-based lifestyles.

In addition to vitamins, moringa is an excellent source of minerals such as calcium, potassium, iron, and magnesium. Calcium and potassium are vital for maintaining healthy bones and regulating blood pressure, respectively. Iron is essential for the production of red blood cells, making moringa an excellent natural remedy for individuals dealing with anemia or looking to enhance their overall energy levels. This mineral-rich profile is particularly beneficial for vegetarians and vegans, who may struggle to obtain adequate amounts of these nutrients from their diets.

The protein content in moringa is another notable feature, as it contains all nine essential amino acids, making it a complete protein source. This characteristic is especially valuable for those adhering to plant-based diets, where protein sources can sometimes be limited. Incorporating moringa into meals can significantly contribute to daily protein requirements while also providing a range of other health benefits. The presence of antioxidants in moringa, including quercetin and chlorogenic acid, further enhances its nutritional value, offering protective effects against chronic diseases.

Moreover, the health benefits of moringa extend beyond mere nutrition. Its anti-inflammatory properties can aid in reducing the risk of chronic conditions, making it an effective natural remedy for various ailments. Traditional medicine practices have utilized moringa for centuries, recognizing its potential to support digestive health, enhance metabolic functions, and promote overall wellness. As research continues to unveil the myriad benefits associated with moringa, its role in holistic health becomes increasingly prominent.

For parents and caregivers, incorporating moringa into family diets can be an excellent way to ensure children receive essential nutrients necessary for growth and development. Moringa supplements, powders, and teas can easily be integrated into meals, offering a convenient option for busy lifestyles. As academics and researchers delve deeper into the nutritional and medicinal properties of moringa, its potential impact on health and wellness will likely continue to gain attention, further solidifying its status as a vital component of sustainable nutrition and natural healing practices.

Overview of Moringa's Benefits

Moringa, often referred to as the "miracle tree," has garnered significant attention for its extensive range of health benefits, making it a staple in the diets of health enthusiasts and wellness seekers alike. Rich in essential nutrients, Moringa leaves are packed with vitamins A, C, and E, as well as a host of minerals such as calcium, potassium, and iron. These components contribute to its reputation as a superfood, providing a powerful boost to the immune system, improving overall energy levels, and supporting metabolic health. Furthermore, the presence of antioxidants in Moringa plays a crucial role in combating oxidative stress, thereby reducing the risk of chronic diseases.

In addition to its nutritional profile, Moringa has a long history of use in traditional medicine practices. Various cultures have utilized its roots, leaves, and pods for their therapeutic properties. Moringa is known for its anti-inflammatory effects, which can alleviate conditions such as arthritis and joint pain. Moreover, its natural antibacterial and antifungal properties make it an effective remedy for infections. For parents and caregivers, incorporating Moringa into children's diets can help enhance their growth and development, thanks to its rich amino acid content and essential vitamins.

The beauty benefits of Moringa oil are also noteworthy, particularly for those interested in natural skincare. Moringa oil is lightweight and absorbs easily, making it an ideal moisturizer that nourishes the skin without clogging pores. Its anti-aging properties, derived from antioxidants and fatty acids, help maintain skin elasticity and promote a radiant complexion. This makes it a popular choice among those seeking vegan and vegetarian-friendly beauty products. Furthermore, the oil's antimicrobial properties can aid in treating skin conditions, thereby positioning Moringa as a versatile ingredient in herbal remedies and natural healing.

Beyond personal health, Moringa's impact on the environment cannot be overlooked. As a fast-growing tree that thrives in arid conditions, Moringa plays a significant role in combating climate change. Its ability to sequester carbon makes it an effective tool in reducing greenhouse gases in the atmosphere. Additionally, Moringa cultivation supports soil health and prevents erosion, promoting sustainable agricultural practices. For academics and researchers, these environmental benefits present a rich area of study, highlighting the intersection of nutrition, health, and ecological sustainability.

Finally, Moringa's versatility extends to pet health and nutrition, where it can be an excellent supplement for dogs and other animals.

Packed with nutrients that support immune function and overall vitality, Moringa can enhance the diets of pets, particularly those on raw or vegetarian diets. Its inclusion in pet food can lead to healthier skin, a shinier coat, and improved digestion. In summary, the myriad benefits of Moringa—from its nutritional and medicinal properties to its environmental significance—position it as a vital component of a sustainable wellness lifestyle, appealing to a diverse audience committed to health and ecological stewardship.

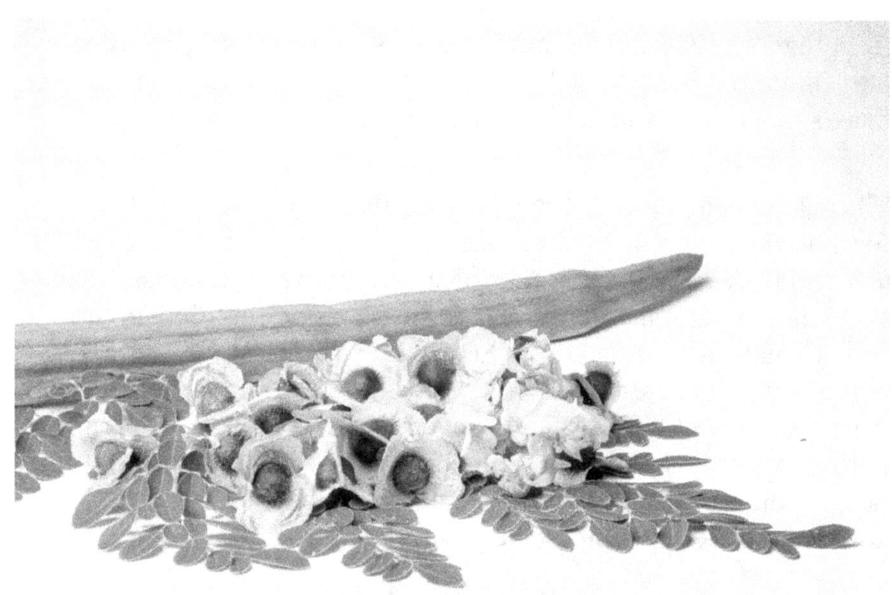

Chapter 2: Moringa: The Miracle Tree

Nutritional Benefits

Moringa, often referred to as the "Miracle Tree," boasts an impressive nutritional profile that positions it as a powerful ally for those committed to health and wellness. Rich in essential vitamins and minerals, moringa leaves are particularly high in vitamin A, vitamin C, potassium, calcium, and iron. This diverse nutrient content makes moringa an excellent addition to vegan and vegetarian diets, providing essential nutrients that are sometimes lacking in plant-based eating. For health enthusiasts and fitness seekers, incorporating moringa can enhance energy levels and overall vitality, supporting both physical performance and recovery.

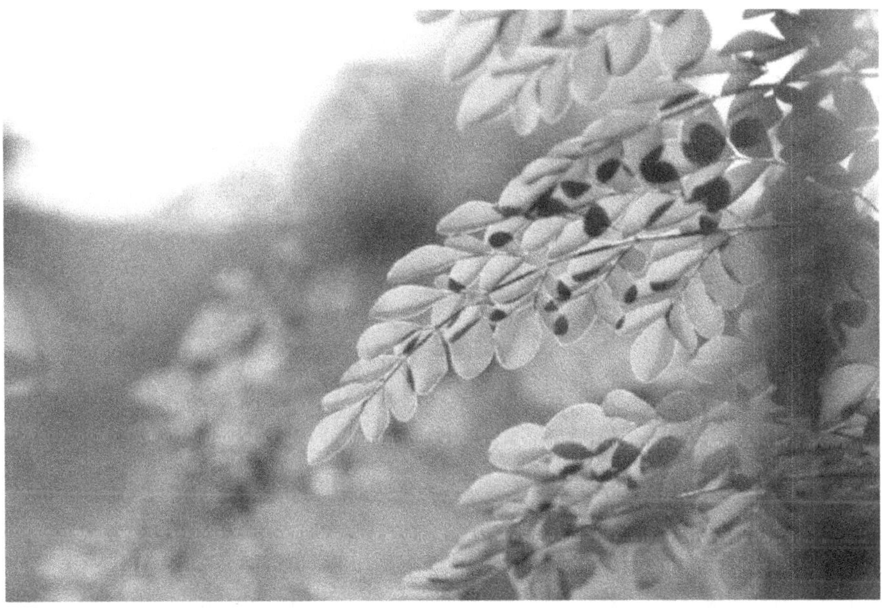

One of the standout features of moringa is its high antioxidant content. Antioxidants play a crucial role in combating oxidative stress and inflammation, which are linked to numerous chronic diseases. Moringa leaves contain quercetin, chlorogenic acid, and beta-carotene, among other powerful antioxidants. These compounds help protect the body from free radical damage, making moringa a valuable resource for natural remedy users looking to bolster their immune system and overall health. Regular consumption of moringa can contribute to a more resilient body and help maintain optimal health.

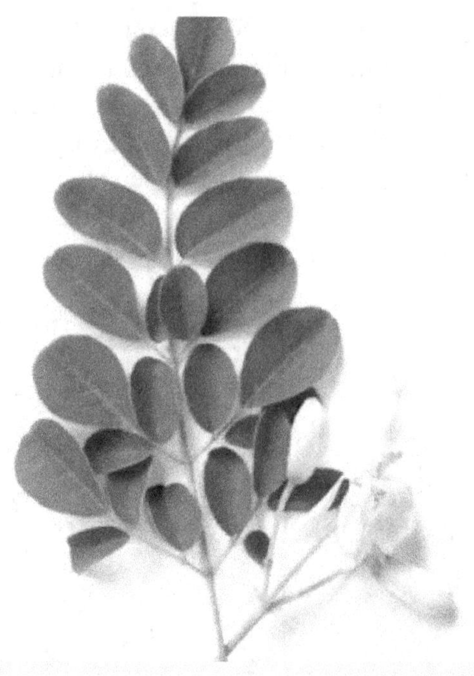

Moreover, moringa is a rich source of protein, providing all nine essential amino acids. This makes it an exceptional choice for vegetarians and vegans who may struggle to meet their protein needs through traditional plant sources. The protein content in moringa can support muscle repair and growth, making it an ideal supplement for fitness enthusiasts. Additionally, moringa's amino acids are vital for various bodily functions, including the production of enzymes and hormones, thus underscoring its role in a balanced diet.

Parents and caregivers can also benefit from introducing moringa into their family's diet. The nutritional benefits of moringa can support healthy growth and development in children. Its iron content is particularly beneficial for preventing anemia, a common concern in young populations. Moringa can be easily incorporated into various meals, from smoothies to soups, ensuring that children receive essential nutrients in a palatable form. By educating families about moringa's benefits, caregivers can promote healthier eating habits that last a lifetime.

For academics and researchers, the exploration of moringa's nutritional benefits opens avenues for further investigation into its role in public health and sustainability. Understanding its nutrient density and potential applications in food security and nutrition can lead to innovative solutions for addressing malnutrition, particularly in developing regions. Research into moringa not only highlights its benefits for individual health but also its potential contributions to broader environmental and social challenges. As interest in sustainable wellness grows, moringa stands out as a key player in nurturing both human health and the health of our planet.

Medicinal Properties

Moringa, often referred to as the "Miracle Tree," boasts a wealth of medicinal properties that have been cherished in traditional medicine for centuries. Its leaves, seeds, and pods are packed with essential nutrients, including vitamins A, C, and E, which play a crucial role in antioxidant activity, protecting the body from oxidative stress. In addition to these vitamins, moringa contains significant amounts of calcium, iron, and potassium, making it a valuable dietary supplement for those seeking to enhance their overall health. Regular consumption of moringa can support immune function, improve digestion, and contribute to maintaining healthy blood sugar levels, addressing various health concerns that are prevalent in today's society.

The anti-inflammatory properties of moringa are particularly noteworthy, as chronic inflammation is linked to numerous health issues, including heart disease and diabetes. Moringa contains compounds such as isothiocyanates and flavonoids, which have been shown to inhibit inflammatory pathways in the body. This natural anti-inflammatory effect can be beneficial for individuals suffering from conditions like arthritis or other inflammatory disorders. By integrating moringa into their diets, health enthusiasts can harness its potential to reduce inflammation and promote better joint and overall body health.

Moringa's role in traditional medicine practices is well-documented across various cultures. In Ayurvedic medicine, for instance, moringa is revered for its ability to balance the body's doshas, promoting harmony between physical and mental health. It is often used to treat ailments such as respiratory disorders, digestive issues, and skin conditions. Similarly, in African and Asian cultures, moringa has been employed as a remedy for malnutrition, particularly among children, due to its rich nutrient profile. The versatility of moringa in treating diverse health problems underscores its importance as a natural remedy and highlights its potential as a sustainable solution to health challenges faced by many communities.

The benefits of moringa extend beyond individual health, as its medicinal properties can also contribute to community wellness. By promoting the cultivation and consumption of moringa, communities can address issues of malnutrition and food insecurity. Moringa's ability to thrive in arid conditions makes it a sustainable crop that can be grown in regions where other food sources may be scarce. This not only supports local economies but also empowers individuals to take charge of their health through accessible nutrition. For parents and caregivers, incorporating moringa into family meals can encourage healthier eating habits while ensuring that children receive essential nutrients for growth and development.

Research continues to explore the full extent of moringa's medicinal benefits, with ongoing studies investigating its potential in areas such as cancer prevention and cardiovascular health. For academics and researchers, moringa presents an intriguing subject for further exploration, particularly in the context of developing natural remedies that can complement conventional medical treatments. As interest in plant-based solutions grows among fitness and wellness seekers, moringa stands out as a prime candidate for inclusion in holistic health regimens. By unlocking the medicinal properties of this remarkable tree, individuals can embrace a more sustainable approach to health and well-being, while contributing to environmental conservation and community resilience.

Environmental Benefits

Moringa, often referred to as the "miracle tree," is not only a powerhouse of nutrition and medicinal properties but also offers significant environmental benefits that resonate with health enthusiasts and those committed to sustainable living. One of the most prominent advantages of cultivating moringa is its ability to improve soil health. Moringa trees have deep root systems that help prevent soil erosion and promote soil fertility. Their leaves, rich in nitrogen, can be used as green manure, enriching the soil and supporting the growth of other plants. This symbiotic relationship enhances agricultural practices, especially in regions prone to soil degradation.

Furthermore, moringa trees play a vital role in mitigating climate change. They are known for their high carbon sequestration potential, absorbing significant amounts of carbon dioxide from the atmosphere. By planting moringa on a larger scale, communities can contribute to reducing greenhouse gases, thereby combating global warming. This makes moringa not only a beneficial crop for personal health and wellness but also a strategic ally in the fight against environmental degradation. The tree's ability to thrive in arid conditions means it can be cultivated in areas where other crops may fail, providing a sustainable source of nutrition while helping to restore ecological balance.

In addition to its role in carbon sequestration, moringa's cultivation promotes biodiversity. The tree attracts various beneficial insects and birds, which contribute to the overall health of the ecosystem. By creating habitats for pollinators and other wildlife, moringa cultivation encourages a diverse range of species. This biodiversity is essential for resilient ecosystems, which can better withstand environmental stresses and contribute to sustainable agricultural practices. For parents and caregivers, planting moringa can be an educational opportunity, teaching children about the importance of biodiversity and the interconnectedness of all living things.

Moreover, moringa is an efficient crop that requires minimal water compared to many traditional agricultural plants. Its drought-resistant nature makes it an ideal choice for areas facing water scarcity, ultimately promoting sustainable agricultural practices in regions where water conservation is crucial. For vegans and vegetarians, the ability to cultivate moringa in diverse climates allows for a sustainable source of plant-based nutrition, reducing reliance on industrial farming methods that often contribute to environmental degradation. This aligns with the values of those seeking to minimize their ecological footprint while maintaining optimal health.

Lastly, the environmental benefits of moringa extend to its potential in natural pest control and organic farming. Moringa leaves and seeds have been shown to possess insecticidal properties, which can reduce the need for chemical pesticides in agricultural practices. This aligns with the growing trend among health enthusiasts and natural remedy users who advocate for chemical-free living. By incorporating moringa into agricultural systems, farmers can promote healthy ecosystems while providing nutritious food, thereby enhancing both personal wellness and environmental sustainability. As more individuals and communities recognize these benefits, the cultivation of moringa can become a cornerstone of sustainable practices for future generations.

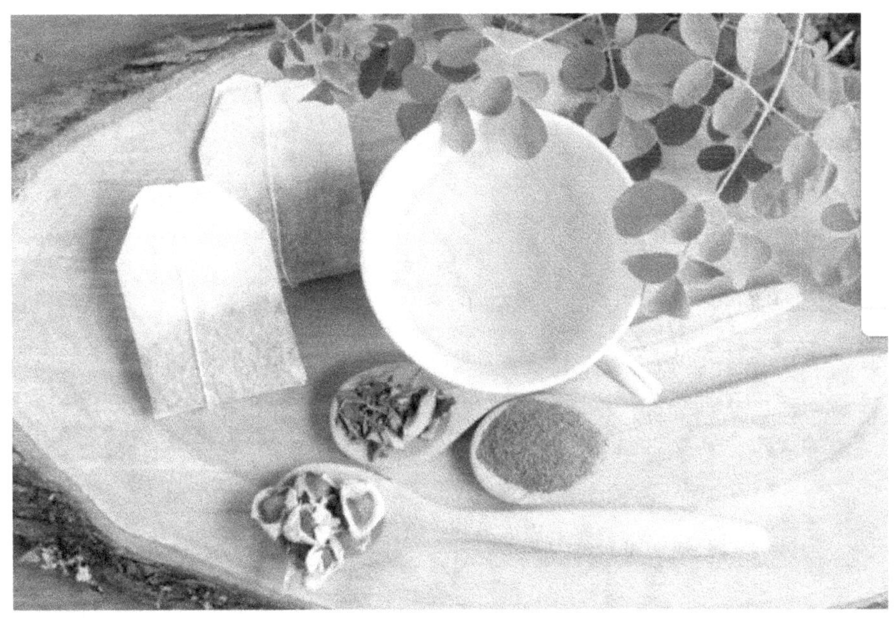

Chapter 3: Moringa in Traditional Medicine Practices

Historical Uses of Moringa

Moringa, often referred to as the "miracle tree," has a rich history that spans various cultures and regions. Its leaves, seeds, and pods have been utilized for centuries across Africa, Asia, and Latin America, showcasing its adaptability and importance in traditional medicine. Ancient civilizations recognized the nutritional and medicinal properties of moringa, often using it as a food source and a remedy for various ailments. Historical texts indicate that in regions such as India, the leaves were consumed to enhance energy levels and overall health, while in Africa, the plant has been employed to combat malnutrition and boost immunity.

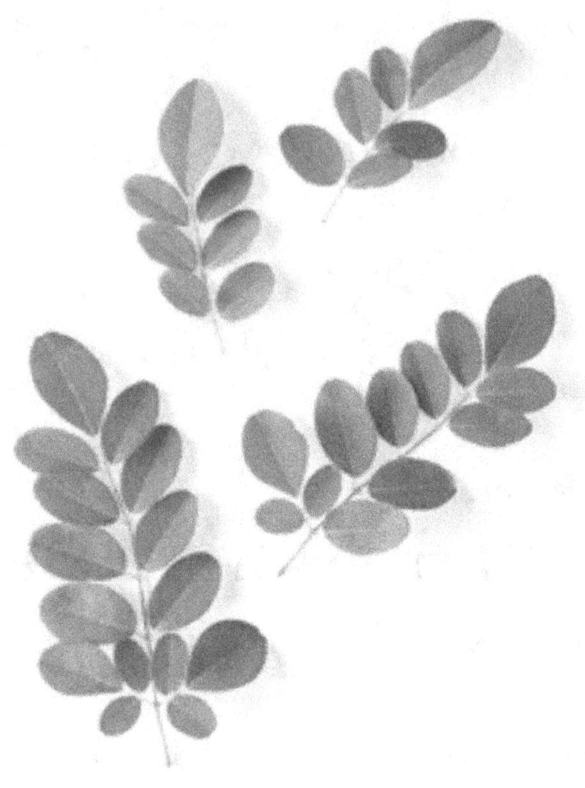

In traditional medicine practices, moringa has played a crucial role in treating a range of conditions. Ayurvedic medicine, a holistic healing system from India, has long utilized moringa for its anti-inflammatory, antioxidant, and antibacterial properties. Practitioners have recommended moringa for digestive issues, respiratory problems, and skin conditions, making it a staple in herbal remedies.

Similarly, in African communities, the roots and bark have been used to prepare potions and poultices for various ailments, demonstrating the tree's versatility as a resource for natural healing.

Moringa oil, extracted from the seeds, has also found its place in historical beauty rituals and skincare. Known for its moisturizing and nourishing qualities, this oil has been used by various cultures for centuries to enhance skin health and manage hair conditions. Its high levels of oleic acid make it a popular choice for cosmetic formulations, and traditional practices often included its application to promote radiance and combat dryness. The historical use of moringa oil highlights the tree's significance not only in nutrition but also in beauty and personal care.

The environmental benefits of moringa have also been recognized throughout history. Its fast growth and ability to thrive in arid conditions have made it a valuable asset in sustainable agriculture. In many regions, moringa is planted to combat soil erosion and improve soil fertility, which is essential for maintaining ecological balance. The tree's capacity for carbon sequestration plays a vital role in climate change mitigation efforts. Historical usage patterns indicate that communities have long understood the importance of integrating moringa into their agricultural practices to enhance resilience against environmental challenges.

In contemporary times, the legacy of moringa's historical uses continues to influence modern health and wellness trends. As health enthusiasts, fitness seekers, and natural remedy users rediscover the benefits of this remarkable plant, its applications in nutrition, personal care, and environmental sustainability gain renewed attention. The ongoing exploration of moringa's potential underscores its significance as a multifaceted resource, bridging traditional wisdom with contemporary wellness practices. By understanding its historical context, we can appreciate the enduring value of moringa in promoting health and sustainability.

Cultural Significance

The cultural significance of moringa extends deeply into various communities around the world, where it has been utilized not only for its nutritional benefits but also for its medicinal properties and ecological impact. In many traditional societies, moringa serves as a vital source of sustenance and healing. Its leaves, seeds, and pods have been integrated into daily diets and traditional medicine, showcasing a profound understanding of its health benefits. This relationship between culture and moringa emphasizes the importance of conserving such indigenous practices while promoting sustainable wellness.

In regions like South Asia and Africa, moringa is often referred to as a "miracle tree" due to its versatility and resilience. Local communities have relied on moringa as a food source rich in vitamins, minerals, and proteins. The leaves are commonly cooked in stews or dried and powdered for use in various recipes, highlighting their role in enhancing food security. Additionally, traditional healers incorporate moringa into their remedies for ailments ranging from inflammation to malnutrition, demonstrating a holistic approach to health that resonates with contemporary wellness philosophies.

The beauty benefits of moringa oil have also made it culturally significant, particularly in regions where natural beauty products are preferred over synthetic options. Moringa oil is celebrated for its moisturizing properties and high antioxidant content, making it a popular ingredient in skincare and hair care routines. This cultural embrace of natural beauty remedies aligns with the growing trend among health enthusiasts and wellness seekers who prioritize organic and sustainable products, reinforcing the idea that ancient practices can inform modern lifestyles.

Moringa's environmental significance further enhances its cultural importance, especially in discussions on climate change and sustainability. As communities face the impacts of environmental degradation, moringa presents an opportunity for reforestation and carbon sequestration. The tree's rapid growth and ability to thrive in arid conditions make it a valuable resource for combating soil erosion and enhancing biodiversity. This ecological role is increasingly recognized by academics and researchers looking to integrate traditional knowledge with scientific approaches to sustainability.

Lastly, the cultural significance of moringa extends to its use in pet health and nutrition. As awareness of holistic pet care grows, many pet owners are turning to natural remedies, including moringa, to support their animals' health. The inclusion of moringa in pet diets highlights a shift towards more informed and health-conscious decisions, reflecting a broader cultural movement that values natural solutions for overall wellness. Through these various lenses, moringa emerges not only as a nutritional powerhouse but also as a symbol of sustainable living deeply rooted in cultural practices.

Modern Applications in Traditional Medicine

Modern applications in traditional medicine have increasingly integrated the wisdom of age-old practices with contemporary scientific understanding. Moringa oleifera, often referred to as the "miracle tree," exemplifies this synergy. Traditional systems of medicine, such as Ayurveda and Traditional Chinese Medicine, have long recognized the therapeutic potential of Moringa leaves, seeds, and pods. Today, health enthusiasts and wellness seekers are rediscovering these components not just for their nutritional value but also for their diverse health benefits. Research has expanded to validate and explore the efficacy of Moringa in managing conditions like diabetes, hypertension, and inflammation, bridging the gap between ancient knowledge and modern medical practices.

The use of Moringa in traditional medicine extends beyond nutrition; its applications in herbal remedies and natural healing are noteworthy. Traditional healers have employed Moringa for its anti-inflammatory, antioxidant, and antimicrobial properties, which are now being substantiated by scientific studies. This validation is crucial for natural remedy users who seek evidence-based options for health management. Moringa's rich profile of vitamins, minerals, and phytochemicals supports its role in enhancing immune function and promoting overall wellness, making it a staple in many natural remedy formulations today.

Moreover, Moringa oil has gained significant traction in the beauty and personal care industry, transcending its roots in traditional practices. The oil, extracted from Moringa seeds, boasts moisturizing and nourishing properties that align with the growing demand for natural beauty products. Vegan and vegetarian consumers are particularly drawn to Moringa oil as a sustainable alternative to synthetic ingredients. Its applications range from skin care to hair care, affirming the tree's versatility and relevance in modern wellness regimes. The intersection of traditional knowledge and contemporary beauty trends illustrates how Moringa continues to inspire innovative approaches to self-care.

The environmental benefits of Moringa also play a critical role in its modern applications. As concerns about climate change and sustainability intensify, Moringa's ability to thrive in challenging conditions and its contributions to carbon sequestration have garnered attention from academics and researchers. Integrating Moringa cultivation into sustainable agricultural practices not only promotes biodiversity but also supports food security. This dual focus on health and environmental stewardship empowers individuals and communities to adopt Moringa as a viable solution for enhancing both personal wellness and ecological health.

Finally, the incorporation of Moringa into pet health and nutrition further exemplifies its relevance in contemporary wellness discussions. Pet owners are increasingly seeking natural dietary supplements for their animals, recognizing the importance of holistic approaches to pet care. Moringa's nutrient-dense profile can benefit pets by supporting their immune systems and overall vitality. As more research emerges on the safe application of Moringa in animal nutrition, caregivers can make informed decisions that align with their values of health and sustainability, ensuring that both people and pets thrive in harmony with nature.

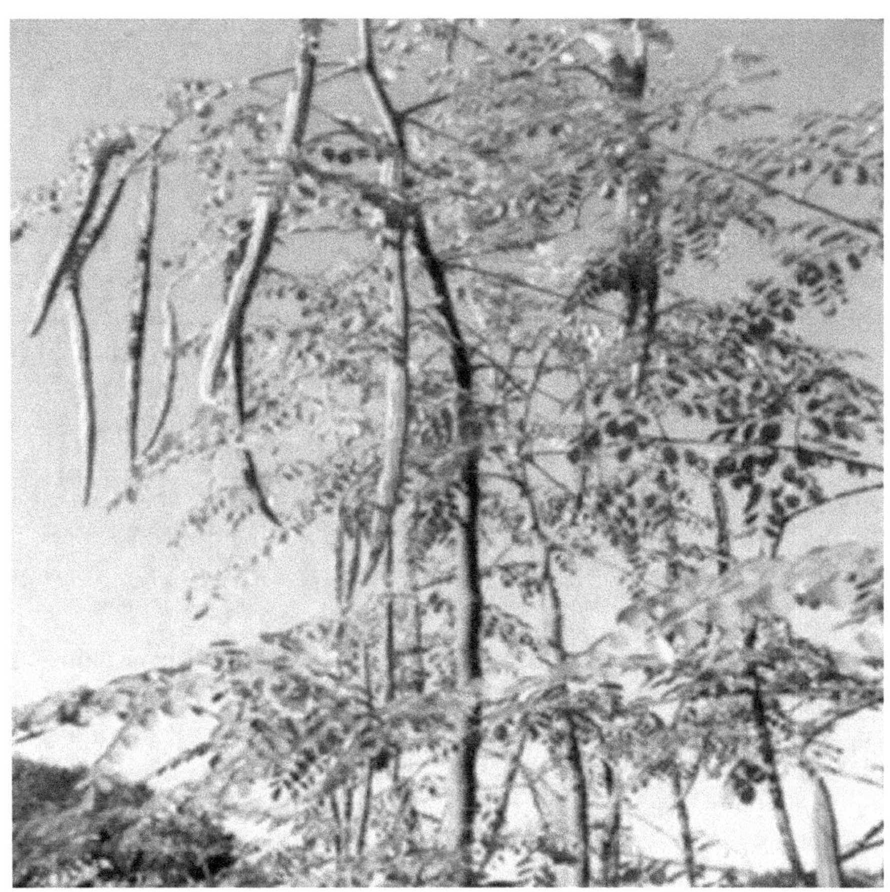

Chapter 4: Moringa Oil and Its Beauty Benefits

Extraction and Production

Moringa, often referred to as the "Miracle Tree," has gained significant attention for its diverse applications in health and wellness. The process of extraction and production of moringa products is vital to harnessing its full potential. Harvesting begins with the leaves, which are the most nutrient-dense part of the tree. These leaves are typically collected by hand, ensuring minimal disruption to the tree's growth. After harvesting, the leaves are washed to remove any dirt or contaminants and then dried, either in the sun or through artificial means. This drying process is crucial, as it preserves the nutritional content while preventing spoilage.

Once dried, the moringa leaves can be ground into a fine powder, which is a popular form for consumption. This powder retains a high concentration of vitamins, minerals, and antioxidants, making it an ideal supplement for individuals seeking to enhance their diets. The production of moringa powder often involves careful monitoring of temperature and humidity during the drying process to ensure that the nutrients remain intact. This attention to detail in the extraction process not only maximizes the health benefits but also ensures that the product meets the standards required by health enthusiasts and wellness seekers.

In addition to the leaves, moringa seeds also hold significant value. Moringa seeds can be pressed to extract oil, which is rich in oleic acid and has numerous beauty benefits. The extraction of moringa oil involves cold pressing, a method that preserves the oil's nutritional and therapeutic properties. This oil is increasingly used in cosmetic formulations for its moisturizing and anti-aging effects. As consumers become more aware of the benefits of natural ingredients, the demand for moringa oil has risen, prompting producers to adopt sustainable practices that ensure the continued health of moringa trees and the surrounding ecosystems.

Sustainability is a critical consideration in the extraction and production of moringa products. Many producers are adopting agroforestry systems that integrate moringa cultivation with other crops, promoting biodiversity and soil health. These practices not only enhance the yield of moringa but also contribute to the fight against climate change through carbon sequestration. By planting moringa trees, farmers can improve their land's resilience against climate impacts while providing a valuable resource for nutrition and wellness. This approach aligns with the goals of health enthusiasts who prioritize ecological health alongside personal well-being.

As research into moringa's benefits continues to expand, the importance of responsible extraction and production methods cannot be overstated. Academics and researchers are increasingly focusing on the environmental impacts of moringa cultivation, including its role in sustainable agriculture and its potential in herbal remedies. The commitment to sustainable practices ensures that moringa remains a viable resource for future generations, benefiting not only health enthusiasts and natural remedy users but also the planet as a whole. By understanding the extraction and production processes, consumers can make informed choices that support their health goals while contributing to environmental sustainability.

Skin Care Applications

Skin care applications of moringa have garnered significant interest among health enthusiasts and those seeking natural remedies. Moringa, often referred to as the miracle tree, is packed with a plethora of nutrients, antioxidants, and anti-inflammatory properties that make it a valuable ingredient in skin care formulations. The leaves, seeds, and oil of moringa can be utilized in various ways to enhance skin health, addressing common concerns such as dryness, aging, and blemishes. By incorporating moringa into daily routines, individuals can benefit from its rich profile and nurture their skin naturally.

Moringa oil, derived from the seeds of the tree, is particularly lauded for its moisturizing and nourishing properties. This lightweight oil is easily absorbed by the skin, making it an excellent natural moisturizer that does not clog pores. Rich in oleic acid, moringa oil helps to hydrate and soothe the skin, promoting a supple and radiant complexion. Additionally, its high concentration of antioxidants, including vitamins A and C, assists in combating free radicals, which can lead to premature aging. Regular application of moringa oil can help improve skin elasticity and reduce the appearance of fine lines, aligning with the goals of fitness and wellness seekers who prioritize healthy aging.

In traditional medicine practices, moringa has been used for centuries to treat various skin ailments. Its antimicrobial properties make it effective in addressing common issues such as acne and other skin infections. The antibacterial and antifungal qualities of moringa can help cleanse the skin and prevent breakouts, making it a preferred choice for those who lean towards natural remedies. Moreover, moringa's anti-inflammatory effects can alleviate irritation and redness, providing relief for sensitive skin. This holistic approach to skin care resonates well with vegans and vegetarians, who often seek plant-based solutions to enhance their beauty routines.

The environmental benefits of moringa also extend to its role in sustainable skin care. As a fast-growing, drought-resistant tree, moringa can be cultivated in various climates, contributing to local economies and reducing the carbon footprint associated with conventional beauty products. By choosing moringa-based skin care options, consumers can support eco-friendly practices that prioritize sustainability. This aligns seamlessly with the values of academics and researchers who study the impact of natural ingredients on both health and environmental well-being, emphasizing the importance of responsible sourcing and production in the beauty industry.

For parents and caregivers, moringa offers a safe and effective option for nurturing the delicate skin of children. Its gentle properties make it suitable for various skin types, including sensitive and dry skin often seen in younger individuals. Moringa-infused creams and balms can provide essential nutrients and hydration without the harsh chemicals often found in conventional products. As more families turn to natural healing practices, incorporating moringa into skin care routines not only supports skin health but also promotes a lifestyle that values sustainability and wellness, making it a cherished addition to any household.

Hair Care Benefits

Moringa, often celebrated for its impressive nutritional profile, extends its benefits to hair care, making it a valuable addition to the routines of health enthusiasts and natural remedy users alike. Rich in vitamins A, C, and E, as well as essential fatty acids, moringa oil and leaves provide nourishment that promotes healthy hair growth. These nutrients strengthen hair follicles, reduce breakage, and enhance overall hair texture. For those in the vegan and vegetarian communities, integrating moringa into hair care regimens offers a plant-based solution to maintaining luscious locks without the use of synthetic chemicals.

The moisturizing properties of moringa oil are particularly beneficial for individuals with dry or damaged hair. Its high oleic acid content allows it to penetrate the hair shaft more effectively than many conventional oils, delivering deep hydration. This moisture retention not only helps to combat frizz but also adds shine and softness to the hair. Parents and caregivers can utilize moringa oil as a natural conditioner, ensuring that children's hair remains healthy and manageable without exposing them to harmful ingredients found in many commercial products.

In addition to providing moisture, moringa also boasts antimicrobial properties that can address common scalp issues such as dandruff and irritation. The antioxidants found in moringa help to combat oxidative stress on the scalp, promoting a healthier environment for hair to grow. For fitness and wellness seekers, maintaining a healthy scalp is just as important as overall body wellness, as a clean and well-nourished scalp contributes to the vitality of hair growth and retention.

The role of moringa in traditional medicine practices further underscores its significance in hair care. Many cultures have employed moringa for centuries not only for its nutritional benefits but also for its topical applications. Herbalists often recommend moringa-infused oils and masks as natural treatments for various hair ailments. This historical context enriches the understanding of moringa's role in wellness, demonstrating its time-honored effectiveness in promoting healthy hair naturally.

Finally, the environmental benefits of moringa cultivation cannot be overlooked in the discussion of its hair care advantages. As a sustainable crop, moringa trees contribute to soil health and biodiversity, making them an ideal choice for eco-conscious consumers. By choosing moringa-based hair care products, individuals not only invest in their personal health but also support sustainable agricultural practices. This alignment with environmental values resonates with academics and researchers interested in the intersection of natural health and ecological responsibility, reinforcing the importance of sustainable wellness in every aspect of life.

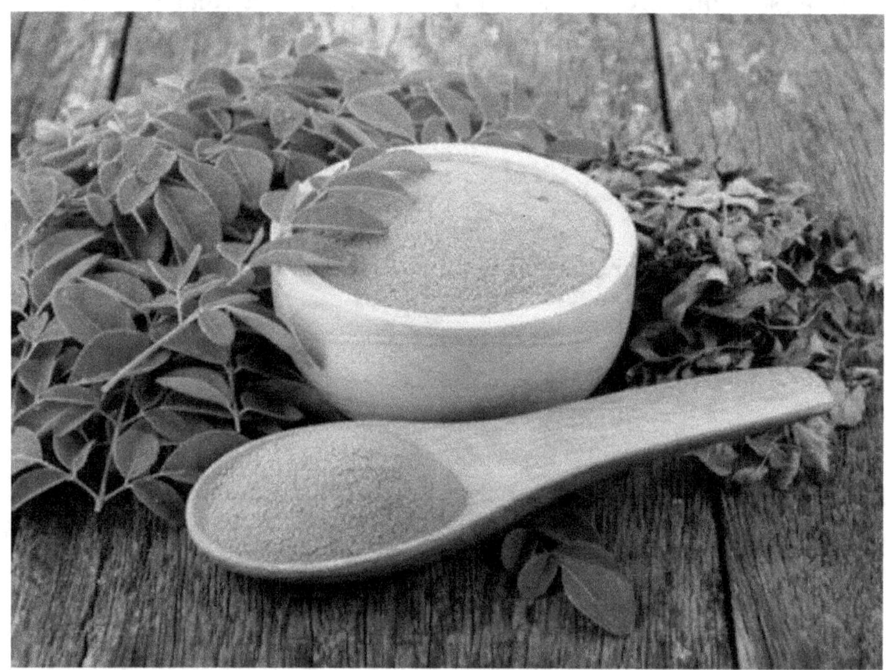

Chapter 5: Moringa's Impact on Climate Change and Carbon Sequestration

Understanding Climate Change

Climate change represents one of the most pressing challenges facing our planet today, with far-reaching implications for health, agriculture, and the environment. It is primarily driven by the increase in greenhouse gas emissions resulting from human activities, such as burning fossil fuels, deforestation, and industrial processes. These activities have led to a rise in global temperatures, disrupted weather patterns, and an increase in the frequency of extreme weather events. Understanding the science behind climate change is crucial for health enthusiasts, fitness seekers, and natural remedy users, as these changes can impact food security, nutritional quality, and overall well-being.

The consequences of climate change extend beyond environmental degradation; they also pose significant risks to human health. Rising temperatures can exacerbate respiratory and cardiovascular conditions, while changing weather patterns can disrupt food supply chains, leading to malnutrition and foodborne illnesses. For parents and caregivers, the health of their children is particularly vulnerable to these changes. Extreme heat, poor air quality, and increased prevalence of vector-borne diseases such as malaria and dengue fever can threaten the health of future generations. Thus, understanding climate change is vital for making informed choices about health and wellness.

One of the key environmental strategies to combat climate change lies in carbon sequestration, the process of capturing and storing atmospheric carbon dioxide. Moringa, often referred to as the "Miracle Tree," plays a significant role in this process due to its rapid growth and resilience. By cultivating moringa trees, we can enhance soil quality, prevent erosion, and sequester carbon effectively. This makes moringa not only a nutritional powerhouse but also an environmentally friendly crop that contributes to climate resilience. For vegans, vegetarians, and those seeking natural remedies, integrating moringa into their diets can promote both personal health and environmental sustainability.

Furthermore, traditional medicine practices that incorporate moringa highlight its dual benefits for health and the environment. Many cultures have utilized various parts of the moringa tree for their medicinal properties, from leaves to seeds and oil. By promoting the use of moringa in herbal remedies and natural healing, we can foster a deeper connection between health and environmental stewardship. This approach aligns with the values of academics and researchers who seek to explore sustainable practices that address both human health and ecological balance.

In summary, understanding climate change is essential for individuals invested in their health and well-being. By recognizing the interplay between environmental factors and personal health, we can make choices that support sustainable practices. Moringa offers an exemplary model of how a single plant can contribute to both health and environmental goals. Embracing moringa not only enhances our nutritional intake but also fosters a more sustainable future, illustrating the vital link between personal wellness and the health of our planet.

Moringa's Role in Carbon Sequestration

Moringa, often referred to as the "Miracle Tree," plays a significant role in carbon sequestration, a process crucial for mitigating climate change. Carbon sequestration involves capturing and storing atmospheric carbon dioxide, reducing greenhouse gas concentrations. Moringa trees are particularly effective in this regard due to their rapid growth and extensive root systems. These roots not only stabilize soil but also enhance its nutrient content, thereby supporting a healthier ecosystem. By cultivating Moringa, individuals can contribute to a natural solution for carbon capture, aligning their health and wellness pursuits with environmental sustainability.

The unique biology of Moringa makes it an excellent candidate for carbon sequestration. Its leaves, which are rich in nutrients, grow densely and can absorb significant amounts of carbon dioxide during photosynthesis. Studies have shown that Moringa can sequester carbon at a rate comparable to or even exceeding that of other tree species. This remarkable capability is vital as the world grapples with rising CO2 levels. For health enthusiasts and those invested in natural remedies, understanding Moringa's environmental benefits offers an additional layer of motivation for incorporating this nutrient-dense plant into their diets and practices.

Moreover, the cultivation of Moringa has additional environmental benefits that extend beyond carbon sequestration. By planting Moringa trees, communities can improve soil health, reduce erosion, and increase biodiversity. The tree's ability to thrive in various climates and soil conditions makes it a valuable resource for reforestation efforts in degraded areas. For parents and caregivers, promoting Moringa not only benefits their families nutritionally but also fosters a sense of responsibility towards environmental stewardship. This dual approach emphasizes the interconnectedness of health and ecological well-being.

The role of Moringa in combating climate change is particularly relevant for academics and researchers focused on sustainable practices. Ongoing research into the carbon sequestration capabilities of Moringa trees is crucial for developing effective climate strategies. Investigating the optimal planting methods, growth conditions, and potential integration into agroforestry systems can enhance our understanding and application of Moringa in carbon management. This knowledge not only contributes to academic discourse but also empowers communities to actively participate in sustainability efforts.

In conclusion, Moringa's role in carbon sequestration presents a compelling narrative for those pursuing health and environmental benefits. By embracing Moringa as a dietary staple and an ecological ally, individuals can take actionable steps toward improving their well-being while also contributing to the health of the planet. As the awareness of Moringa's potential grows, it becomes clear that this remarkable tree is not only a source of nutrition and natural remedies but also a key player in the fight against climate change, making it an invaluable asset for a sustainable future.

Sustainable Farming Practices

Sustainable farming practices are essential for enhancing the health of our planet and the well-being of its inhabitants. These practices prioritize ecological balance and the responsible use of resources, which is particularly significant when considering crops like Moringa, often referred to as the "miracle tree." By adopting methods such as crop rotation, organic farming, and permaculture, farmers can cultivate Moringa while maintaining soil fertility, reducing pest infestations, and minimizing chemical inputs. This approach not only supports the growth of Moringa but also contributes to a healthier ecosystem that benefits health enthusiasts and wellness seekers who prioritize sustainable and clean nutrition.

One of the key components of sustainable farming is the use of organic fertilizers and natural pest control methods. These techniques are crucial in Moringa cultivation, as they reduce dependency on synthetic chemicals that can harm both human health and the environment. By utilizing compost, cover crops, and integrated pest management strategies, farmers can create a biodiverse environment that encourages beneficial organisms. This not only leads to healthier Moringa plants but also ensures that the nutritional content remains intact, appealing to vegans, vegetarians, and natural remedy users who seek high-quality, chemical-free food sources.

Water conservation is another critical aspect of sustainable farming practices. Efficient irrigation techniques, such as drip irrigation and rainwater harvesting, can significantly reduce water usage while still providing adequate moisture to crops. Given Moringa's resilience in arid conditions, farmers can implement these strategies to cultivate this nutrient-rich plant in regions with limited water resources. By promoting water-efficient farming, we can help mitigate the impact of climate change and support communities in adapting to changing environmental conditions, ultimately benefiting parents, caregivers, and health-conscious individuals who rely on Moringa for its extensive health benefits.

Agroforestry is an innovative sustainable farming practice that integrates trees, such as Moringa, into agricultural systems. This method not only enhances biodiversity but also improves soil health and reduces erosion. Moringa's deep root system can help sustain soil moisture and prevent land degradation, making it a valuable asset in sustainable farming. Furthermore, the presence of Moringa trees can provide shade and improve crop yields in companion planting scenarios. For academics and researchers, understanding the dynamics of such practices can yield insights into sustainable agriculture's role in combating climate change and promoting environmental health.

Finally, community engagement and education play a vital role in the success of sustainable farming practices. Farmers who are informed about the environmental and health benefits of Moringa can adopt and advocate for sustainable methods more effectively. Workshops, local farming initiatives, and partnerships with health organizations can foster a culture of sustainability among consumers and producers alike. By promoting awareness of Moringa's environmental impact and its nutritional value, we can empower communities to support sustainable farming practices that benefit not only individual health but also the planet as a whole. This collective effort is essential in the journey towards a healthier future for all.

Chapter 6: Moringa for Pet Health and Nutrition

Nutritional Benefits for Pets

Moringa, often referred to as the "miracle tree," is celebrated for its rich nutritional profile, not just for human consumption but also for the health of our pets. The leaves, seeds, and pods of the Moringa tree are packed with essential vitamins, minerals, and amino acids, making them an excellent addition to pet diets. Incorporating Moringa into pet food can help enhance overall health, bolster the immune system, and contribute to a longer, healthier life for our animal companions.

One of the significant nutritional benefits of Moringa for pets is its high content of vitamins A, C, and E. These vitamins are crucial for maintaining a healthy immune system and promoting skin and coat health. Pets that receive adequate amounts of these vitamins are less susceptible to infections and skin conditions, which can often lead to discomfort and health complications. Additionally, the antioxidant properties of Moringa help combat oxidative stress in pets, further supporting their overall vitality.

Moringa also contains essential fatty acids and protein, which play vital roles in the growth and repair of tissues. For active pets, these nutrients are particularly important as they help maintain muscle mass and promote recovery after exercise. Moringa's protein content offers a complete amino acid profile, making it a valuable supplement for both dogs and cats, especially those on vegetarian or vegan diets. By ensuring that pets receive sufficient protein through plant-based sources, caregivers can support their pets' health while aligning with their own dietary values.

The anti-inflammatory properties of Moringa are another noteworthy benefit. Conditions such as arthritis or joint pain are common in aging pets, and incorporating Moringa into their diet may provide relief from these ailments. The natural compounds found in Moringa can help reduce inflammation, thus improving mobility and quality of life for senior pets. This aspect makes Moringa not only a nutritional powerhouse but also a potential natural remedy to alleviate chronic pain in pets.

In conclusion, Moringa offers a myriad of nutritional benefits that can significantly enhance the health and well-being of pets. As health enthusiasts and caregivers seek natural and holistic approaches to pet nutrition, Moringa stands out as a sustainable option that aligns with the principles of wellness and environmental responsibility. By integrating this superfood into pet diets, caregivers can ensure that their furry friends receive the essential nutrients they need while promoting a healthier planet.

Medicinal Uses for Common Pet Ailments

Moringa, often referred to as the "miracle tree," has garnered attention not only for its nutritional and environmental benefits but also for its potential in promoting pet health. Many common ailments that afflict our beloved pets, such as skin irritations, digestive issues, and joint pain, can be addressed through natural remedies, with moringa being a key component. This subchapter delves into the medicinal uses of moringa for common pet ailments, providing health enthusiasts and caregivers with valuable insights into how this remarkable plant can support the well-being of their furry companions.

Skin issues are prevalent among pets, often manifesting as itching, redness, or inflammation. Moringa leaves are rich in antioxidants and anti-inflammatory properties, making them a beneficial addition to a pet's diet or topical applications. The leaves can be ground into a powder and mixed with water to create a paste that can be applied to irritated areas, providing soothing relief. Additionally, moringa oil, extracted from the seeds, is known for its emollient properties, which can help moisturize dry skin and support overall skin health. By incorporating moringa into their routines, pet owners can promote healthier skin and reduce the need for pharmaceutical interventions.

Digestive problems, such as diarrhea or constipation, are commonly experienced by pets and can lead to discomfort and more serious health issues. Moringa is a natural source of dietary fiber, which can help regulate digestion and promote gut health. Including moringa powder in a pet's food can enhance their diet with essential nutrients while aiding in digestive regularity. Furthermore, the anti-inflammatory properties of moringa can soothe gastrointestinal irritation, making it a gentle yet effective remedy for digestive upsets. Caregivers can take comfort in knowing that moringa offers a holistic approach to managing their pets' digestive health.

Joint pain and mobility issues are significant concerns, especially for older pets or those with existing health conditions. Moringa's anti-inflammatory characteristics can play a vital role in alleviating pain and improving joint function. By incorporating moringa into their diet, pet owners may help reduce inflammation and enhance mobility in their pets. Additionally, moringa is rich in essential amino acids, calcium, and other nutrients that contribute to bone health. For pets suffering from arthritis or general stiffness, moringa can serve as a natural supplement to support their overall musculoskeletal health.

As awareness of the benefits of natural remedies continues to grow, many pet owners are seeking alternatives to conventional treatments. Moringa stands out as a versatile and beneficial addition to pet care regimens, offering solutions for common ailments while aligning with holistic health principles. For health enthusiasts and caregivers who prioritize natural approaches, understanding the applications of moringa can empower them to make informed choices for their pets' health. By embracing the potential of this remarkable tree, they can foster a sustainable wellness journey for both themselves and their furry friends, nurturing a bond that thrives on health and vitality.

Incorporating Moringa into Pet Diets

Incorporating Moringa into pet diets can significantly enhance the nutritional value of the food we provide to our furry companions. Moringa, often referred to as the "miracle tree," boasts a comprehensive profile of vitamins, minerals, and antioxidants that can benefit animals just as much as they benefit humans. This superfood is rich in essential amino acids, vitamins A, C, and E, calcium, and iron, making it an excellent addition to the diets of pets, particularly dogs and cats, who thrive on a balanced nutrient regimen.

When introducing Moringa into a pet's diet, it is important to consider the appropriate forms and quantities. Moringa leaves can be dried and powdered, which makes them easy to incorporate into homemade pet food or sprinkled onto commercial kibble. Additionally, Moringa oil can be used as a supplement, providing healthy fats that promote a shiny coat and overall skin health. However, it is crucial to start with small amounts and gradually increase the dosage to prevent gastrointestinal upset, allowing the pet to adjust to this new ingredient.

Moringa's numerous health benefits extend to pets as well. Its anti-inflammatory properties may help alleviate conditions such as arthritis in older animals, while its antioxidant content can bolster the immune system, helping pets fend off illnesses. Moreover, Moringa is known to support digestive health, which is particularly beneficial for pets prone to gastrointestinal issues. By enhancing the overall health and vitality of pets, Moringa can contribute to a longer, happier life.

For pet owners interested in natural remedies, Moringa serves as an excellent alternative to synthetic supplements. Many commercially available pet vitamins and supplements can contain fillers and artificial ingredients that may not align with a holistic approach to pet care. In contrast, Moringa is a plant-based option that is safe when introduced appropriately. It not only provides essential nutrients but also supports the environmental sustainability that many health enthusiasts seek in their lifestyle choices.

As more pet owners become aware of the health benefits of natural foods, incorporating Moringa into pet diets aligns with the growing trend of holistic pet care. This incorporation not only enhances pet health but also reflects a commitment to sustainability and responsible sourcing. By choosing Moringa, pet owners can support their pets' well-being while also contributing to the broader

movement towards eco-friendly practices in nutrition, ultimately
benefiting both animals and the planet.

Chapter 7: Moringa in Herbal Remedies and Natural Healing

Overview of Herbal Remedies

Herbal remedies have gained significant attention in recent years as
individuals increasingly seek natural alternatives to conventional
medicine. This shift towards holistic health practices is particularly
relevant among health enthusiasts, fitness seekers, and those who
prioritize plant-based diets. Herbal remedies, derived from various
plants, have been utilized for centuries in traditional medicine
practices across diverse cultures. They offer a rich tapestry of
benefits, making them an essential component of modern wellness
strategies, especially for those keen on sustainable and
environmentally friendly health solutions.

Moringa, often referred to as the "miracle tree," exemplifies the
potential of herbal remedies. Rich in vitamins, minerals, and
antioxidants, Moringa leaves, seeds, and pods are used in a variety of
health applications. This plant not only supports nutritional needs but
also plays a role in addressing various health issues, ranging from
inflammation to digestive problems. By incorporating Moringa into
their diets, individuals can access a natural source of essential
nutrients that promote overall well-being, aligning perfectly with the
values of vegans, vegetarians, and natural remedy users.

In traditional medicine practices, Moringa has been revered for its
therapeutic properties. Many cultures have utilized its leaves and
roots to treat ailments such as respiratory disorders, skin conditions,

and even as a natural energy booster. The knowledge passed down through generations highlights the importance of herbal remedies in maintaining health and preventing disease. For parents and caregivers, understanding these traditional uses can empower them to make informed decisions about incorporating Moringa into their families' diets, fostering a proactive approach to health.

The beauty benefits of Moringa oil further expand its appeal within the realm of herbal remedies. Known for its moisturizing and anti-aging properties, Moringa oil is increasingly used in skincare products. Its high content of oleic acid and antioxidants makes it an excellent choice for nourishing the skin and enhancing its natural glow. This aspect of Moringa resonates with wellness seekers who are interested in natural beauty solutions, providing an opportunity to combine health and aesthetics through the use of plant-based products.

Lastly, the environmental benefits of Moringa cannot be overlooked. As concerns about climate change and sustainability grow, Moringa stands out as a resilient plant that contributes to carbon sequestration and soil health. Its deep root system helps prevent soil erosion, while its fast growth rate allows for quick biomass production. For academics and researchers, studying Moringa's environmental impact offers insights into sustainable agriculture practices that can benefit both human health and the planet. This holistic view of Moringa positions it as not just a herbal remedy but a vital element in the nexus of health, beauty, and environmental stewardship.

Moringa's Role in Natural Healing

Moringa, often referred to as the "Miracle Tree," has garnered attention not only for its impressive nutritional profile but also for its significant role in natural healing practices across various cultures. This remarkable plant, native to parts of Asia and Africa, has a long history of use in traditional medicine, where every part of the tree—from leaves and seeds to roots and flowers—has been utilized for its therapeutic properties. Rich in vitamins, minerals, and antioxidants, moringa is believed to support the body's healing processes, making it a valuable addition to the diets of health enthusiasts and natural remedy users alike.

The leaves of moringa are particularly renowned for their medicinal benefits. They are packed with essential nutrients, including vitamin C, calcium, and potassium, which contribute to overall health. These leaves are often consumed as a powder, in teas, or as fresh foliage in salads. The anti-inflammatory properties of moringa are supported by research, indicating that it may help alleviate conditions such as arthritis and other inflammatory diseases. Additionally, the presence of powerful antioxidants in moringa helps combat oxidative stress, potentially reducing the risk of chronic diseases and supporting longevity.

Moringa's role in traditional medicine extends beyond mere nutrition. In various cultures, it has been used as a natural remedy for ailments ranging from digestive issues to skin conditions. For instance, the seeds of the moringa tree are known for their antibacterial properties and have been used to purify water, highlighting their importance in both health and environmental sustainability. Moreover, moringa oil, extracted from the seeds, is celebrated not only for its culinary uses but also for its benefits in skincare. Its moisturizing properties make it an excellent choice for those seeking natural beauty solutions.

Parents and caregivers can also benefit from incorporating moringa into their families' diets. The nutritional density of moringa makes it an ideal supplement for growing children, providing essential nutrients that support healthy development. Furthermore, its potential to enhance immune function is particularly relevant in today's health-conscious world. By introducing moringa into family meals or offering it in forms like smoothies or snacks, caregivers can promote overall wellness while also instilling healthy eating habits in children.

In the realm of research, ongoing studies continue to explore the vast potential of moringa as a natural healing agent. As academics and researchers delve deeper into its phytochemical properties, there is a growing understanding of how moringa can be integrated into modern healthcare practices. The convergence of traditional knowledge and contemporary scientific inquiry promises to unlock even more benefits of this extraordinary plant, further solidifying its place in the pantheon of natural remedies. As we continue to discover and appreciate the multifaceted uses of moringa, its role in promoting sustainable wellness becomes increasingly clear.

Preparation and Usage of Moringa in Remedies

Moringa, often referred to as the miracle tree, has garnered attention for its diverse applications in remedies and health practices. Preparation of moringa for use in remedies can be straightforward, yet understanding the best methods ensures that one maximizes its nutritional and medicinal benefits. The leaves, pods, seeds, and even the flowers of the moringa tree are rich in vitamins, minerals, and antioxidants, making them valuable in various health applications. The first step in utilizing moringa for remedies involves selecting fresh, organic leaves, which can be consumed raw, cooked, or dried. When preparing dried moringa leaves, they should be air-dried away from direct sunlight to preserve their nutritional value, and can then be ground into a fine powder for easy incorporation into foods or beverages.

One popular method of using moringa is through infusion. To prepare a moringa tea, fresh or dried leaves can be steeped in hot water for several minutes, allowing their nutrients to be extracted. This infusion can serve as a refreshing beverage with numerous health benefits, including anti-inflammatory and antioxidant properties. Additionally, moringa tea can be sweetened with honey or combined with other herbs to enhance flavor and therapeutic effects. For those seeking a more potent remedy, moringa can be blended into smoothies, where its taste can be masked by other ingredients, making it an easy addition to daily diets.

In addition to leaf preparations, moringa seeds hold significant medicinal potential. These seeds can be consumed raw, roasted, or ground into powder. They are known for their antibacterial and anti-inflammatory properties, making them useful in treating various conditions. A common remedy involves soaking the seeds overnight in water to enhance their digestibility and nutrient absorption. Once prepared, they can be added to salads, soups, or smoothies, offering a nutritious boost to any meal. Furthermore, oil extracted from moringa seeds is gaining popularity in the beauty industry, known for its moisturizing and anti-aging properties when applied topically.

Moringa's versatility extends to its use in herbal blends and natural healing practices. It is often combined with other herbs to create powerful tinctures and salves. For those interested in natural remedies, moringa can be incorporated into herbal formulas targeting specific ailments, such as digestive issues, skin irritations, or immune support. When crafting these blends, it is essential to consider the synergistic effects of various herbs, as well as individual health needs. Proper research and consultation with herbalists or health professionals can enhance the efficacy of these remedies.

As interest in sustainable wellness grows, the environmental benefits of moringa also merit consideration. By cultivating moringa, individuals contribute to biodiversity and soil health, while also promoting climate resilience. The tree's ability to sequester carbon and thrive in arid conditions makes it a valuable asset in combating climate change. For health enthusiasts and caregivers, introducing moringa into daily practices not only supports personal well-being but also aligns with environmental sustainability. This holistic approach to health and healing underscores the multifaceted advantages of moringa, establishing it as a cornerstone in both dietary and ecological wellness.

Chapter 8: Incorporating Moringa into Daily Life

Recipes and Dietary Tips

Incorporating moringa into your diet can significantly enhance your nutritional intake while supporting sustainable practices. Moringa leaves are rich in vitamins, minerals, and antioxidants, making them a valuable addition to any meal. One of the simplest ways to enjoy moringa is by adding powdered leaves to smoothies or juices. A combination of spinach, banana, and a teaspoon of moringa powder can create a nutrient-packed drink that boosts energy levels and provides essential nutrients. Additionally, moringa powder can be sprinkled on salads or mixed into dressings to infuse your meals with its unique flavor and health benefits.

For those exploring plant-based diets, moringa serves as an excellent protein source. A delicious recipe involves making moringa-infused quinoa salad. Cook quinoa and mix it with diced vegetables such as bell peppers, cucumbers, and cherry tomatoes. Add a generous handful of fresh moringa leaves, a squeeze of lemon, and a drizzle of olive oil for a refreshing meal that is high in protein and packed with essential amino acids. This salad not only nourishes the body but also highlights the versatility of moringa in everyday meals.

When it comes to cooking with moringa, it is crucial to understand the best methods to preserve its nutritional profile. Steaming or lightly sautéing moringa leaves can retain their beneficial compounds better than boiling. A simple stir-fry with tofu, moringa leaves, garlic, and ginger makes for a quick, nutritious dish that can be served over brown rice or whole grains. This method maximizes the health benefits while providing a satisfying meal that is perfect for busy lifestyles.

In addition to its culinary uses, moringa can be integrated into herbal remedies and natural healing practices. A soothing moringa tea can be made by steeping moringa leaves in hot water, providing a calming drink that supports digestion and hydration. For parents and caregivers, this tea can serve as a natural remedy for minor ailments, highlighting moringa's role in traditional medicine. Furthermore, combining moringa powder with honey and lemon can create a natural immune-boosting syrup, ideal for seasonal wellness.

Lastly, for those concerned about environmental sustainability, using moringa in your dietary practices aligns with eco-friendly habits. Moringa trees are drought-resistant and can thrive in various climates, making them a sustainable crop. By incorporating moringa into your diet, you support agricultural practices that contribute to climate resilience. Sharing recipes and dietary tips centered around moringa not only promotes health but also encourages a broader appreciation for this remarkable plant and its potential to enhance our well-being and the environment.

Moringa Supplements and Products

Moringa supplements and products have gained significant popularity in recent years, reflecting a growing interest in natural health solutions among diverse groups, including health enthusiasts, fitness seekers, and those who adhere to vegan and vegetarian lifestyles. Moringa, often referred to as the "miracle tree," offers a wealth of nutrients, including vitamins A, C, and E, calcium, potassium, and protein. These components contribute to its status as a powerful supplement capable of enhancing overall wellness. Available in various forms such as powders, capsules, teas, and oils, moringa products cater to a range of preferences and health goals, making it accessible for a wider audience.

In traditional medicine, moringa has been used for centuries to address various health concerns. Its roots, leaves, and seeds have been utilized in herbal remedies, providing anti-inflammatory, antioxidant, and antibacterial properties. Research highlights moringa's potential in treating conditions such as diabetes, hypertension, and malnutrition. As more individuals turn to natural remedies, the growing body of scientific evidence supporting moringa's health benefits encourages further exploration into its role in contemporary wellness practices.

For those interested in beauty and personal care, moringa oil has emerged as a popular ingredient in skincare and haircare products. Rich in oleic acid and antioxidants, moringa oil helps to hydrate and nourish the skin while combating signs of aging. Its anti-inflammatory properties make it suitable for sensitive skin, and its ability to promote hair health has captured the attention of beauty enthusiasts seeking natural alternatives. Incorporating moringa oil into daily routines can enhance beauty regimens while aligning with a holistic approach to wellness.

Moringa's environmental benefits further solidify its appeal among sustainability-minded individuals. The tree is known for its ability to thrive in arid conditions, making it an excellent candidate for agroforestry and sustainable agriculture initiatives. Its deep root system helps prevent soil erosion, while its leaves and pods can be harvested without harming the tree, promoting sustainable harvesting practices. Moreover, moringa's capacity for carbon sequestration contributes positively to climate change mitigation efforts, attracting the attention of academics and researchers interested in sustainable solutions for environmental challenges.

As awareness of moringa continues to grow, it invites curiosity about its applications beyond human health. Pet owners are increasingly recognizing the nutritional benefits of moringa for their animals, with its rich vitamin and mineral content supporting overall health and vitality. Moringa's versatility in various forms—such as powders or treats—makes it easy to incorporate into pet diets. This holistic approach to health, integrating moringa for both humans and pets, showcases the broad potential of this remarkable plant, encouraging a deeper exploration of its myriad benefits for individuals, families, and the environment.

Sustainable Sourcing of Moringa

Sustainable sourcing of moringa is essential for ensuring that its cultivation and harvest do not deplete natural resources or harm local ecosystems. Moringa, often referred to as the miracle tree, is celebrated not only for its impressive nutritional profile but also for its adaptability to various climates and soils. Sustainable practices involve growing moringa in a manner that maintains soil health, conserves water, and promotes biodiversity. These practices can include agroforestry systems where moringa trees are integrated with other crops and livestock, creating a symbiotic relationship that enhances soil fertility and reduces the need for chemical fertilizers.

One of the key aspects of sustainable sourcing is the use of organic farming methods. This approach avoids synthetic pesticides and fertilizers that can lead to soil degradation and water pollution. By employing natural pest control measures, such as introducing beneficial insects or using microbial solutions, farmers can protect their moringa crops while maintaining the integrity of the surrounding environment. Furthermore, organic practices often yield higher nutritional quality in moringa leaves and pods, aligning with the health-conscious preferences of vegans, vegetarians, and natural remedy users.

Local sourcing of moringa also plays a crucial role in sustainability. By prioritizing local producers, consumers can reduce their carbon footprint associated with transportation. Additionally, supporting local farmers fosters economic growth in rural communities and encourages the preservation of traditional farming practices. This connection to local agriculture not only enhances the freshness of the moringa products available but also strengthens community ties and promotes cultural heritage, which is particularly important for parents and caregivers seeking healthy options for their families.

Sustainable sourcing practices extend beyond cultivation to include ethical harvesting methods. Responsible harvesting ensures that moringa trees can continue to thrive and regenerate. This involves selecting mature leaves and pods while allowing younger growth to flourish. Educating harvesters about the importance of sustainable techniques can lead to better yields over time and preserve the ecological balance. For academics and researchers, understanding these practices provides valuable insights into sustainable agriculture and its role in combating climate change and promoting health.

Lastly, the impact of moringa on global sustainability cannot be overstated. As a drought-resistant plant, moringa thrives in arid conditions, making it a viable option for regions facing climate challenges. Its ability to sequester carbon further enhances its role in mitigating climate change. By advocating for the sustainable sourcing of moringa, individuals can contribute to a larger movement towards environmental stewardship while reaping the health benefits associated with this remarkable plant. Embracing sustainable practices in moringa cultivation and consumption not only supports personal wellness but also promotes a healthier planet for future generations.

Chapter 9: The Future of Moringa

Research and Innovations

The exploration of Moringa, often referred to as the "Miracle Tree," has become a focal point of research and innovation in both health and environmental sciences. Recent studies have highlighted the remarkable nutritional profile of Moringa leaves, which are rich in essential vitamins, minerals, and antioxidants. Researchers have been examining the potential of Moringa in addressing nutritional deficiencies, particularly in developing regions where malnutrition is prevalent. The findings suggest that incorporating Moringa into daily diets can significantly enhance health outcomes, making it a subject of interest for health enthusiasts and those advocating for plant-based diets.

In the realm of traditional medicine, Moringa has been utilized for centuries, and contemporary research is validating many of these age-old practices. Investigations into its medicinal properties have revealed anti-inflammatory, antimicrobial, and antioxidant effects, contributing to its growing reputation as a natural remedy. This resurgence in interest aligns with the increasing demand for holistic approaches to health, especially among natural remedy users and wellness seekers. Clinical trials and ethnobotanical studies are shedding light on the efficacy of Moringa in treating various ailments, reinforcing its role in the future of integrative medicine.

Moringa oil, derived from the seeds of the tree, has also emerged as a topic of innovative research, particularly in the beauty and personal care industry. Studies are examining the oil's moisturizing properties, its effectiveness as a carrier oil for essential oils, and its potential for promoting skin health. This aligns with the growing trend towards natural and sustainable beauty products among consumers who are increasingly aware of the ingredients in their cosmetics. The exploration of Moringa oil is not only beneficial for individuals seeking organic beauty solutions but also presents opportunities for sustainable sourcing and production practices within the cosmetics industry.

Furthermore, the environmental benefits of Moringa are gaining traction in academic circles, particularly regarding its role in combating climate change and promoting sustainability. Research has demonstrated Moringa's potential for carbon sequestration, which could play a significant role in mitigating global warming. By improving soil health and enhancing biodiversity, Moringa cultivation presents a dual advantage: providing nutritious food while also contributing to environmental restoration. This aspect is particularly appealing to academics and researchers focused on sustainable agriculture and environmental health.

Lastly, the application of Moringa extends beyond human health; it is also being explored for pet nutrition and wellness. Innovative studies are assessing the benefits of Moringa for animal health, focusing on its nutritional content and potential therapeutic properties. This research is vital for pet owners who prioritize natural and holistic diets for their animals. As more evidence emerges regarding Moringa's versatility and efficacy across various domains, it solidifies its status as a multifaceted resource, appealing to a wide audience dedicated to wellness, sustainability, and natural living.

Moringa in Global Health Initiatives

Moringa, often referred to as the "miracle tree," has gained significant recognition in global health initiatives due to its remarkable nutritional and medicinal properties. This plant, native to parts of Africa and Asia, is rich in essential vitamins, minerals, and antioxidants that contribute to overall health and wellness. Health organizations and NGOs have started incorporating moringa into their nutritional programs, particularly in regions facing malnutrition and food insecurity. Its leaves, pods, and seeds are not only edible but also exhibit a high concentration of nutrients that can help combat deficiencies, making moringa an invaluable asset in public health strategies.

The World Health Organization has identified moringa as a potential solution to address micronutrient deficiencies, particularly in developing countries where access to a diverse diet may be limited. The leaves of the moringa tree are a powerhouse of vitamins A, C, and E, as well as calcium and iron. By integrating moringa into school feeding programs and community health initiatives, organizations can improve the nutritional status of vulnerable populations. This approach not only enhances food security but also empowers communities by promoting local agricultural practices that utilize moringa as a sustainable crop.

In addition to its nutritional benefits, moringa has been embraced for its medicinal properties, which have been recognized in various traditional medicine practices. The anti-inflammatory, antimicrobial, and antioxidant properties of moringa have made it a focal point in herbal medicine. Researchers and health practitioners are increasingly exploring the therapeutic potential of moringa in treating chronic conditions such as diabetes, hypertension, and respiratory diseases. This growing interest has led to the development of moringa-based supplements and remedies, offering natural alternatives for individuals seeking holistic health solutions.

The environmental benefits of moringa also align with global health initiatives focused on sustainability. As countries grapple with the challenges of climate change, moringa presents an opportunity for reforestation and biodiversity conservation. Its ability to thrive in arid conditions and improve soil quality makes it an ideal candidate for agroforestry systems, which can enhance food security while sequestering carbon. By promoting moringa cultivation, health initiatives can simultaneously address nutritional needs and environmental concerns, creating a more sustainable future for communities worldwide.

As awareness of moringa's multifaceted benefits continues to spread, health enthusiasts, caregivers, and researchers are encouraged to engage with this remarkable plant. From integrating it into daily diets to exploring its potential in natural remedies, moringa offers a pathway to improved health and wellness. By participating in global health initiatives that prioritize the use of moringa, individuals can contribute to a collective effort toward better nutrition, sustainable agriculture, and environmental stewardship, ultimately fostering a healthier planet for future generations.

The Role of Moringa in Sustainable Development

The role of Moringa in sustainable development cannot be overstated, as it presents a multifaceted approach to addressing both health and environmental challenges. This tree, often referred to as the "miracle tree," is rich in essential nutrients, making it a valuable resource for communities struggling with food insecurity. Moringa leaves are packed with vitamins, minerals, and proteins, which contribute to improved nutrition, especially in regions where malnutrition is prevalent. By integrating Moringa into local diets, communities can enhance their nutritional intake while promoting agricultural diversity and resilience.

In addition to its nutritional benefits, Moringa plays a significant role in traditional medicine practices. Its leaves, pods, and seeds have been utilized for centuries in various cultures for their medicinal properties. By incorporating Moringa into herbal remedies, practitioners can address common health issues naturally, reducing reliance on synthetic medications that may have harmful side effects. This aspect of Moringa not only promotes health and wellness but also aligns with the principles of sustainable development by encouraging the use of locally sourced, natural remedies that support both individual and community health.

The environmental impact of Moringa is equally impressive. This fast-growing tree is known for its ability to thrive in arid conditions, making it an excellent candidate for reforestation and agroforestry projects in areas affected by climate change. Moringa's deep root system helps prevent soil erosion, improves soil fertility, and supports biodiversity. Furthermore, its potential for carbon sequestration helps mitigate the adverse effects of climate change. By planting Moringa, communities can contribute to a healthier ecosystem while simultaneously benefiting from its nutritional and medicinal properties.

Moringa oil has also emerged as a significant player in the beauty and wellness industry, showcasing the tree's versatility. Rich in antioxidants and nutrients, Moringa oil is used in skincare and haircare products, promoting sustainable beauty practices that favor natural ingredients over synthetic alternatives. This shift towards natural beauty products not only aligns with the growing consumer demand for eco-friendly options but also supports sustainable economic development by creating local job opportunities in the cultivation and processing of Moringa.

Lastly, the potential of Moringa extends to pet health and nutrition, offering a holistic approach to animal care. By incorporating Moringa into pet diets, owners can provide their animals with essential nutrients that enhance overall health. This practice emphasizes the interconnectedness of human, animal, and environmental health, embodying the principles of sustainable wellness. As more individuals and communities recognize the comprehensive benefits of Moringa, it becomes clear that this remarkable tree is not only a solution for personal health but also a cornerstone of sustainable development, contributing to a healthier planet for future generations.

Chapter 10: Conclusion

Recap of Moringa's Benefits

Moringa, often referred to as the "Miracle Tree," offers a diverse array of health benefits that make it an invaluable addition to any wellness regimen. Rich in vitamins, minerals, and antioxidants, Moringa leaves are a powerhouse of nutrition. They contain significant amounts of vitamin A, vitamin C, calcium, and iron, making them particularly beneficial for individuals seeking to enhance their dietary intake without relying on synthetic supplements. This nutrient density is especially appealing to health enthusiasts and those following vegan or vegetarian diets, as Moringa provides essential nutrients that are sometimes challenging to obtain from plant-based sources alone.

In addition to its nutritional profile, Moringa has garnered attention for its medicinal properties. Traditional medicine practices have long recognized the therapeutic potential of Moringa, using its leaves, seeds, and pods to treat various ailments. From anti-inflammatory effects to blood sugar regulation, Moringa has been employed in herbal remedies for centuries. Its ability to support immune function and promote overall wellness is particularly relevant for natural remedy users and those interested in holistic health approaches. This ancient wisdom is now being corroborated by modern research, reinforcing Moringa's role as a natural ally in health maintenance.

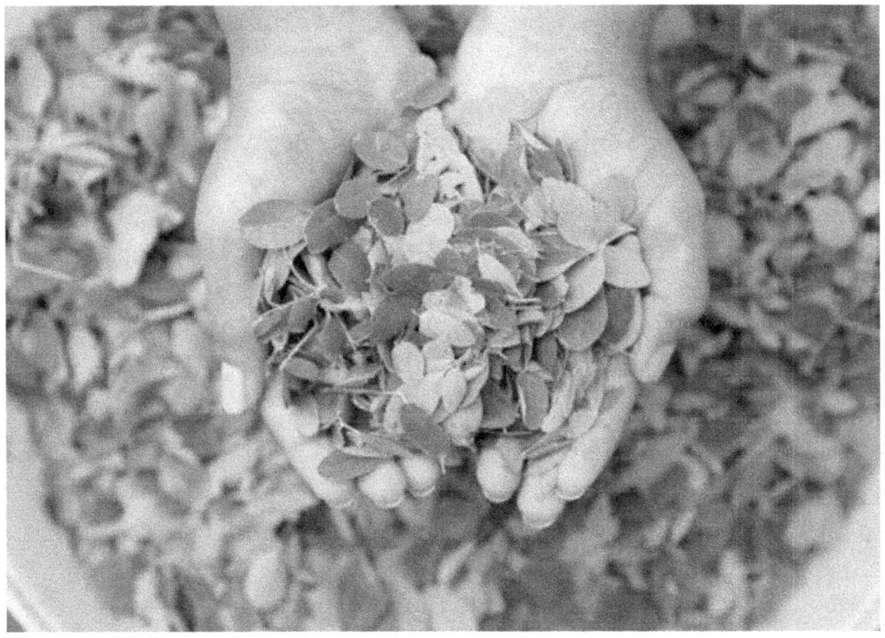

Moringa oil, extracted from the seeds, is another facet of this remarkable plant that contributes to its reputation as a versatile health resource. Rich in oleic acid and antioxidants, Moringa oil is celebrated for its beauty benefits, including skin hydration, anti-aging properties, and its ability to nourish hair. These benefits make it a popular choice among individuals seeking natural skincare and haircare solutions. As consumers increasingly gravitate towards clean beauty products, Moringa oil stands out as an eco-friendly alternative that aligns with a sustainable lifestyle.

Beyond individual health benefits, Moringa plays a crucial role in addressing environmental challenges. Its rapid growth and ability to thrive in arid conditions make it an excellent candidate for promoting sustainable agriculture. Moringa trees contribute to carbon sequestration, helping to mitigate climate change by absorbing carbon dioxide from the atmosphere. For academics and researchers, the exploration of Moringa's environmental impact presents exciting opportunities for sustainable development initiatives. By cultivating Moringa, communities can enhance food security while simultaneously addressing pressing environmental concerns.

Finally, Moringa's benefits extend to pet health and nutrition, offering a holistic approach to caring for our animal companions. Its nutrient profile can support digestion, boost energy levels, and enhance overall vitality in pets. As more pet owners seek natural solutions for their furry friends, Moringa provides a safe and effective option. Whether incorporated into pet food or used as a supplement, Moringa stands out as a plant that nourishes not just human health but the health of our pets, reinforcing the interconnectedness of wellness in all living beings.

Call to Action for Sustainable Practices

In an era where the urgency for sustainable practices has never been more pressing, the integration of Moringa into our daily lives presents a compelling call to action for health enthusiasts and wellness seekers alike. Moringa, often referred to as the "miracle tree," offers a plethora of nutritional and medicinal benefits that not only promote individual health but also contribute positively to environmental sustainability. By embracing Moringa, we can actively participate in a movement that prioritizes wellness for ourselves and the planet.

For fitness and wellness seekers, incorporating Moringa into your diet is a straightforward yet impactful way to enhance your nutritional intake. Rich in vitamins, minerals, and antioxidants,

Moringa leaves can be easily added to smoothies, salads, or even as a supplement. By choosing to integrate such nutrient-dense foods into our lifestyles, we not only nourish our bodies but also support sustainable agricultural practices. Engaging with local farmers who cultivate Moringa organically can further amplify these benefits, fostering community ties and promoting environmentally friendly farming methods.

Vegan and vegetarian communities stand to gain immensely from Moringa's diverse health benefits. As a plant-based source of protein, Moringa can serve as an excellent alternative to animal products, ensuring that nutritional needs are met while adhering to ethical dietary choices. Encouraging the use of Moringa within these diets not only supports individual health but also highlights the importance of plant-based eating in combating climate change. By reducing reliance on resource-intensive animal farming, we can collectively contribute to a more sustainable food system.

Parents and caregivers play a critical role in shaping the dietary habits of future generations. Introducing Moringa into children's diets can instill a sense of appreciation for nutritious foods from a young age. Moreover, its potential benefits for immune support and overall health make it an ideal addition to family meals. By emphasizing the importance of natural remedies and herbal supplements like Moringa, caregivers can equip the next generation with the knowledge and tools necessary to prioritize wellness and sustainability in their own lives.

Academics and researchers have a unique opportunity to explore the myriad benefits of Moringa, both from a health and environmental perspective. By conducting studies on Moringa's role in climate change mitigation, carbon sequestration, and its applications in traditional medicine, scholars can contribute valuable insights to the global conversation on sustainability. Collaboration with practitioners in the field can lead to innovative practices that harness Moringa's potential, thereby driving the momentum towards a healthier, more sustainable future. Engaging in this research not only enriches academic discourse but also empowers communities to make informed decisions that benefit both their health and the environment.

Final Thoughts on Moringa and Wellness

The exploration of Moringa as a pivotal component of wellness encapsulates a multifaceted approach to health that is deeply intertwined with environmental sustainability. As health enthusiasts and wellness seekers, understanding Moringa's rich profile reveals not only its nutritional benefits but also its medicinal properties that have been harnessed in traditional practices for centuries. With its high concentrations of vitamins, minerals, and antioxidants, Moringa stands out as a superfood that can enhance overall well-being, supporting everything from immune function to digestive health. This holistic view positions Moringa as a key player in modern health regimens, appealing to those seeking natural, plant-based solutions.

In the context of traditional medicine, Moringa has held a place of reverence in various cultures, recognized for its ability to address an array of ailments. Its leaves, pods, and seeds have been utilized in herbal remedies that target inflammation, blood sugar regulation, and even malnutrition. The integration of Moringa into contemporary wellness practices reflects a growing appreciation for natural remedies, particularly among vegans and vegetarians who prioritize plant-based nutrition. By bridging the gap between ancient wisdom and modern science, Moringa offers a compelling narrative that resonates with those invested in holistic health approaches.

Beauty and personal care also benefit from Moringa's remarkable properties. Moringa oil, extracted from the seeds, is infused with oleic acid and antioxidants, making it an ideal ingredient for skincare products. Its hydrating and anti-aging effects have garnered attention from beauty enthusiasts and natural remedy users alike. The acknowledgment of Moringa oil's benefits extends beyond topical applications; it embodies the essence of sustainability, as it can be sourced responsibly, aligning with the values of eco-conscious consumers. This intersection of beauty and wellness underscores the versatility of Moringa, enhancing its appeal across diverse demographics.

As the discourse surrounding climate change intensifies, Moringa emerges not just as a health enhancer but also as a champion for environmental health. Its rapid growth and ability to thrive in diverse climates make it a viable option for reforestation and carbon sequestration efforts. By promoting Moringa cultivation, we not only contribute to our own wellness but also take actionable steps toward a healthier planet. This dual benefit speaks to parents and caregivers who seek sustainable choices for their families, creating a legacy of environmental stewardship through mindful consumption.

In sum, the final thoughts on Moringa and wellness converge on a theme of interconnectedness. The nutritional, medicinal, and environmental benefits of Moringa illustrate its potential to transform individual health and contribute positively to global challenges. For academics and researchers, Moringa represents a rich field for further exploration, inviting studies that may unlock even deeper insights into its applications. As we embrace Moringa in our lives, we participate in a larger movement that champions sustainable wellness, fostering a future where personal health and ecological vitality coexist harmoniously.

www.ingramcontent.com/pod-product-compliance
Lightning Source LLC
Chambersburg PA
CBHW051708250726
48653CB00007B/2911